KETO CO(

FOR BEGINNERS

QUICK AND SMART RECIPES TO LOSE WEIGHT AND MAINTAIN YOUR KETOGENIC DIET

DAN BALTWIN

TABLE OF CONTENT

Introduction

Nowadays most people eat too many sugar-based foods. Every day there is more and more evidence that sugar and sweets are bad for us. Unlike other short-lived fad diets, the ketogenic diet has been around for more than ninety years as it was first used to treat patients who suffered from epilepsy. Today, it is also used for weight loss To switch to a ketogenic diet, you must eliminate all processed sugars from your diet . in such a way the body is pushed to the state of ketosis wherein it uses up fat bodies called ketones as its main source of energy instead of glucose. such a way that es up fat bodies called ketones as its main source of energy instead of glucose. You are about to discover a great and very nutritious diet that has changed millions of people's lives. A lifestyle that will fascinate you and make you a new person in no time The ketogenic diet contains moderate carbohydrates. People who follow the ketogenic diet limit the intake of carbohydrates to around 20 to 30 net grams daily or 5% of the daily diet. Net grams refer to the number of carbohydrates that remain after subtracting the grams of dietary fiber. The presence of a higher amount of protein pushes the body to the process called gluconeogenesis wherein protein is converted into glucose. If this happens, the body is not pushed to a state of ketosis. This is the reason why it is so crucial to consume more fat under the ketogenic diet than protein Learning about it is the first and one of the most important things to do now. During this diet, your body will produce less insulin and glucose through the keto diet. Ketosis is a natural process that occurs when we eat less food than usual. The body will quickly adapt to this condition, and you will be able to lose weight in a short time. Your blood sugar will improve, and you will not be prone to diabetes. Your cholesterol levels will improve, and you will feel good right away, what it sounds like. The ketogenic diet is simple and easy to follow if you follow a few simple rules. People usually enter the state of ketosis after 3 to 4 days of consuming little amounts of carbohydrates You don't need to make significant changes, but you do need to know a few things. So, if you want to change your diet and stay healthy, the ketogenic diet is a good choice for you no matter what time of year. In this e-book, you will discover some of the tastiest and easy-to-make recipes. However, the most important thing to remember when starting a ketogenic diet is consistency. Of course, it can sometimes be difficult for you to decline a fraudulent meal when the opportunity presents itself. On vacation or traveling with friends. Is your body is perfectly able to recover after returning to your diet? Then it is essential to keep it as close as possible so that your body maintains a high metabolism. Congratulations on making a life-changing decision! Join the many people like you. Both have adopted a healthier lifestyle and enjoy...

Ketogenic Recipes for Breakfast

Butter Eggs

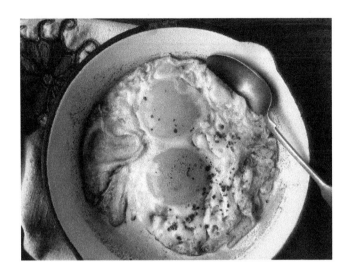

Prep time: 13minutes

Cook time: 15minutes

Servings: 4

Ingredients: 1 teaspoon garlic powder 2 tablespoons butter 1 teaspoon ground paprika 6 eggs, hard-boiled

Method: Peel and cut the eggs into halves. Then melt butter in the skillet and add egg halves and roast them for 1 minute. Sprinkle the eggs with garlic powder and ground paprika.

Nutritional info per serve: Calories 149, Fat 8.6, Fiber 0.3, Carbs 1.3, Protein 8.6

Tasty Poached Eggs

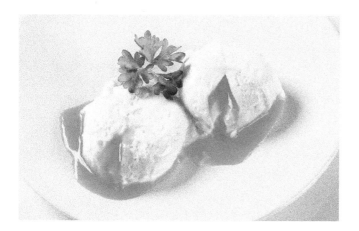

Prep time: 12minutes

Cook time: 38 minutes

Servings: 4

Ingredients: 1 Red bell pepper, chopped   1 spoon paprika   3 garlic cloves, minced 1 tablespoon ghee 1 Serrano pepper, diced 3 tomatoes, diced 1 spoon cumin ¼ spoon chili powder Salt and black pepper 1 tablespoon cilantro, chopped   6 eggs 1 white onion, chopped

Method: Warm-up your skillet with the ghee at medium heat, adds onion, stir and keep for almost 10 minutes. Now, add Serrano pepper and garlic, stir and leave for 1 minute. And then add red bell pepper, stir and cook for 10 minutes. Add tomatoes, cumin, salt, pepper, chili powder, and paprika, stir and cook for 10 minutes. Beat eggs to the pan, season them with pepper & salt, cover the pan and cook for 6 minutes more. Spatter cilantro at the end and distribute to the consumers. Finally enjoy your dish!

Nutritional info per serve: Calories 300, Fat 12, Fiber 3.4, Carbo 22, Protein 14

Morning Granola

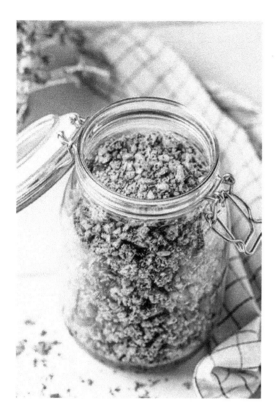

Prep time: 15 minutes

Cook time: 1 hour

Servings: 6

Ingredients: 1 tbsp coconut oil ⅓ cup almond flakes ½ cup almond milk ½ tbsp liquid stevia 1/8 tsp salt 1 tsp lime zest ½ tsp ground cinnamon ½ cup pecans, chopped ½ cup almonds, slivered 2 tbsp pepitas 3 tbsp sunflower seeds ¼ cup flax seeds Preheat the oven to 300°F.

Method: Set a deep pan over medium heat and warm the coconut oil. Add almond flakes and toast for about 2 minutes. Stir in the remaining ingredients. Lay the mixture in an even layer onto a baking sheet lined with a parchment paper. Bake for 1 hour, making sure that you shake gently in intervals of 15 minutes. Serve alongside additional almond milk.

Nutritional info per serve: Kcal 262; Fat: 24.3g, Net Carbs: 9.2g, Protein: 5.1g

Crispy Stuffed Bacon Cups

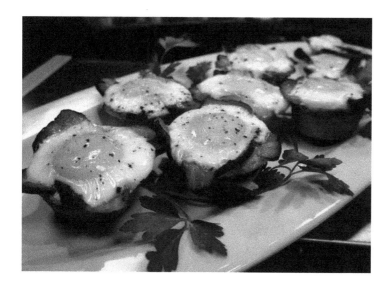

Prep time :10 min

Cook time: 20 min

Servings:12

Ingredients 12 slices bacon 8 eggs 2 oz. red bell pepper, finely diced 2 oz. green bell pepper, finely diced 2 oz. yellow onion, finely diced 5 oz. shredded cheddar cheese 2 tbsp heavy whipping cream 3 tsp extra-virgin olive oil Salt and pepper

Methods: Preheat the oven to 350°F. Line a slice of bacon around the edges of a muffin tin (12 cups) Bake for 12 minutes or until browned. Add the eggs, heavy whipping cream, red and green bell peppers, and onion in a bowl and whisk to combine. Heat olive oil in a pan and cook eggs over low heat until cooked through. Add egg and bell pepper mixture in bacon cups. Top with cheddar cheese. Add to oven and broil until cheese has a nice crust. Remove from the oven and serve.

Nutritional info per serve: Kcal 109 / Fat 12 g. / Carbs 1 g./Pro 5g

Almond Coconut Oatmeal

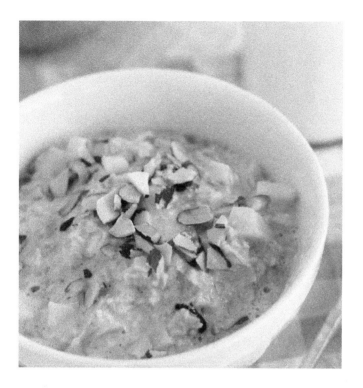

Prep: 5 min

Cook Time: 10 min

Servings: 2

Ingredients: 2 eggs 1 cup almond milk 2 tbsp coconut flour 2 tbsp unsweetened shredded coconut 2 tbsp almond butter

Methods: Add eggs, almond milk, coconut flour in a bowl and whisk together. Heat the mixture in a pot, stir frequently and cook until thickened. Add almond butter to taste. Sprinkle the shredded coconut and serve

Nutritional info per serve: Kcal 253 / Fat 20 g. / Carbs 8 g./Pro 8g.

Blueberry Hemp Seed dish

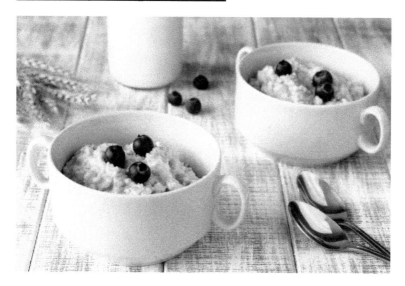

Prep time: 5min

Cook Time: fifteen min

Servings: two

Ingredients: sixteen oz. almond milk eight oz. hemp seeds eight oz. blueberries two tbsp ground flax seeds two tbsp chia seeds two tsp flavourer two tbsp oil

Methods: Add all of the ingredients in a very pot aside from the blueberries. mix and stir well and produce to a boil. Once it's boiling bring down the warmth to a low-medium. permit the dish to simmer for three minutes. Once the mixture has thickened up take away it from the warmth. Transfer the dish into a bowl and add oil and blend well. place the blueberries on high.

Nutritional information per serve: Kcal 265 / Fat 25 gr. / Carbs:7,5gr./Pro2gr

Smoked Salmon Breakfast

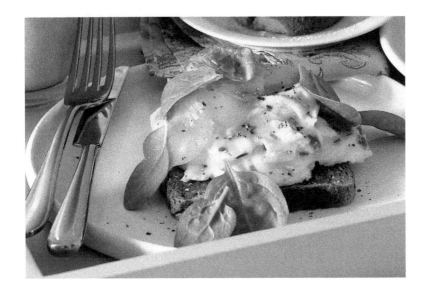

Prep time: 6 minutes

Cook time: 10 minutes

Servings: 3

Ingredients: 4 eggs whisked, ½ teaspoon avocado oil, 4 ounces smoked salmon, chopped. For the sauce: 1 cup coconut milk, Salt ½ cup cashews, soaked, drained, ¼ cup green onions, 1 teaspoon garlic powder, Black pepper, 1 tablespoon lemon juice

Methods: Take your blender, mix cashews with coconut milk, garlic powder, and lemon juice and blend well. Combine salt, pepper, and green onions, blend again well, transfer to a bowl and keep in the fridge for now. Whisk the egg a bit and cook until they are almost done. Inject in your preheated oven and cook until eggs set. Separate eggs on plates, top with smoked salmon, and serve with the green onion sauce on top. Enjoy your recipe!

Nutritional info per serve Kcal 200/ Fat 10/Carbs 11/Pro15g

Sausage Sandwich

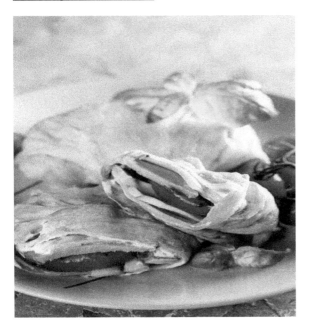

Prep time: 13 minutes

Cook time: 16 minutes

Servings: 4

Ingredients: 4 eggs, 1 tablespoon butter, 1 teaspoon ground black pepper, 8 lettuce leaves, 4 sausages

Methods: Toss the butter in the pan and melt it. Crack the eggs inside and add sausages. Close the lid and cook the ingredients for 5-8 minutes. Then put the eggs and sausages on the lettuce leaves.

Nutritional info per serve: Calories 135, Fat 8.2, Fiber 0.2, Carbs 1, Protein 8.2

Feta and Asparagus Delight

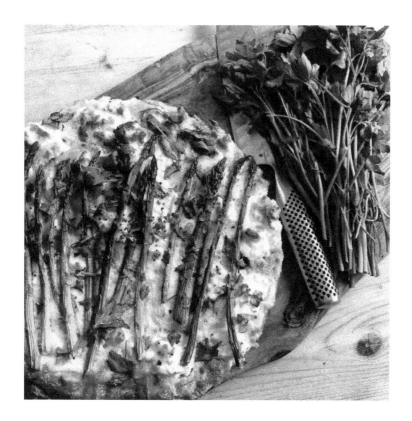

Prep time: 10 minutes

Cook time: 25 minutes

Servings: 2

Ingredients: 12 asparagus spears, olive oil 1tablespoon, 2 green onions, black pepper, 1 garlic clove minced , 6 eggs, Salt, feta cheese (½ cup)

Methods: Warm a pan with some water covering moderate heat, add asparagus, boil for 8 minutes, drain well, chop two spears, and reserve the rest. Heat the pan in oil at medium heat, and add garlic, chopped asparagus, and onions, stir, and cook for 5 minutes. Then Add eggs, pepper, and salt stir, cover, and heat for 5 minutes. Arrange the whole asparagus on top of your frittata, sprinkle cheese, and bake for almost 9 minutes. Distribute among plates & enjoy. Enjoy your breakfast!

Nutritional info per serve: Calories 340/ Fat 12/ Fiber 3/ Carbs 8/ Protein 26

Breakfast Muffins

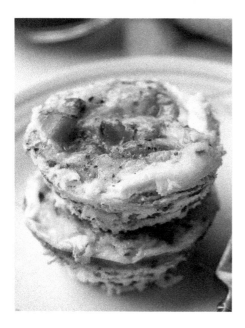

Prep time: 12 min

Cook Time: 35 min

Servings: 10

Ingredients: 4 tbsp butter 4 bacon strips, chopped 10 eggs 2 oz. milk 4 oz. coconut flour 4 oz. chopped baby Spinach 4 oz. ricotta 5 tbsp pesto sauce salt and ground black pepper

Methods: Preheat the oven to 375°F (190°C). Grease muffin cups with butter. Add bacon in a saucepan over medium heat. Stir occasionally until bacon is crisp. Transfer to a plate and set aside. Spray a standard 10 muffin cups with cooking spray and set aside. Add milk, and coconut flour in a large bowl and crack an egg to combine. Season with salt and pepper. Add spinach and bacon and stir to mix. Divide among muffin cups and top with ricotta and pesto. Transfer to oven and bake for about 15 minutes and serve.

Nutritional info per serve: Kcal 92/ Fat 57 g./Carbs 1 g./Protein 6 g.

Chocolate Almond Butter Oatmeal

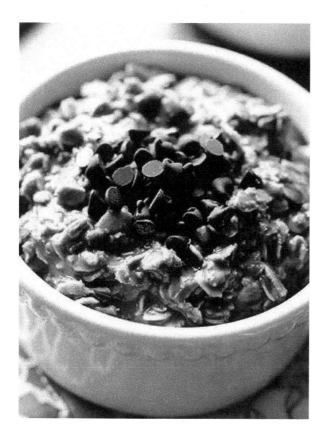

Prep time: 5 min

Cook Time: 10 min

Servings: 2

Ingredients: 4 oz. hemp seeds, 2 tbsp flaxseed meal, 1 tbsp chia seeds, 8 oz. almond milk, 2 tbsp almond butter, 2 tbsp dark chocolate chips

Methods: Add hemp, flaxseed and chia seeds in a saucepan and mix well. Add cream and almond milk and whisk until smooth. Simmer for about 3 minutes over low heat or until thickened, stirring frequently. Stir in almond butter and simmer for 2 minutes and stir in chocolate chips. Let warm before serving.

Nutritional info per serve: Kcal 542/Fat 41g./Carbs 10 g./ Protein 17 g.

Mushroom Scramble

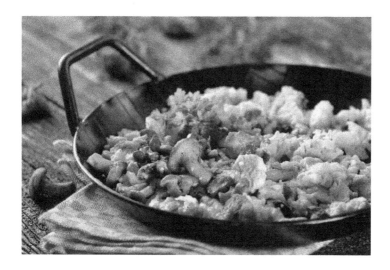

Prep time: 12 minutes

Cook time: 16 minutes

Servings: 2

Ingredients: 1 cup cremini mushrooms, chopped 5 eggs, beaten 2 tablespoons butter 1 teaspoon salt ½ teaspoon ground black pepper

Method: Put butter in the pan and melt it. Add mushrooms, salt, and ground black pepper. Roast the mushrooms for 5-10 minutes on medium heat. Then add beaten eggs and carefully stir the mixture. Cook the scramble for 3 minutes

Nutritional info per serve: Calories 270, Fat 14.9, Fiber 0.4, Carbs 2.7, Protein 14.9

Ketogenic Recipes for lunch

<u>Special Lunch Burgers</u>

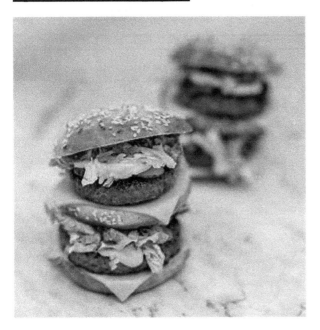

Prep time: 8 minutes

Cook time: 25 minutes

Servings: 7

Ingredients: 1 pound brisket, ground 1 pound beef, ground Salt Black pepper 8 butter slices 1 tablespoon garlic, minced 1 tablespoon Italian seasoning 2 tablespoons mayonnaise 1 tablespoon ghee 2 tablespoons olive oil 1 yellow onion, chopped 1 tablespoon water

Method: In a bowl, mix brisket with beef, salt, pepper, Italian seasoning, garlic, and mayo and stir well. Shape eight patties and make a pocket in each. Stuff each burger with a butter slice and seal. Heat a pan with the olive oil over medium heat, add onions, stir and cook for 2 minutes. Add the water, stir and gather them in the corner of the pan. Place burgers in the pan with the onions and cook them over medium- low heat for 10 minutes. Flip them, add the ghee and cook them for 10 minutes more. Divide burgers on buns and serve them with caramelized onions on prime. Finally, Enjoy!

Nutritional info per serve: KCal: 200/Fat: 8 g/ Pro: 14 g Carbs: 3 gr

Chicken salad

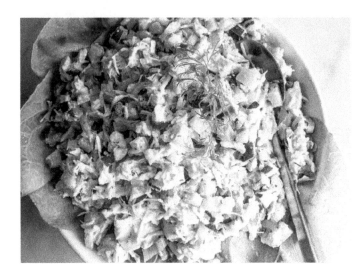

Prep time : 12 minutes

Cook time: 30 minutes

Servings: 5

Ingredients: chicken breast 1 lbs, 3 celery stalks, diced, ½ C Paleo Mayonnaises, 2 teaspoons brown mustard , ½ teaspoon salt, 2 tablespoon Dill, fresh, chopped, ¼ C Pecans, chopped

Methods: On a baking sheet, line the bottom with parchment paper. Preheat the oven to 450 degrees Fahrenheit. heat the kitchen appliance to 450 degrees Fahrenheit. Bake the chicken for concerning quarter-hour or till done through. whereas the chicken is baking, in a bowl, mix the celery, mayonnaise, mustard, and Salt. Place in the fridge to stay cool. take away the chicken from the kitchen appliance once done cookery and chop into bite-sized chunks. enable to chill and so combine into the bowl with the opposite ingredients. It is best to cool overnight in the fridge; however, if you can, eat it immediately. Before serving, top with chopped dill and pecans. Finally, enjoy.

Nutritional info per serve: Kcal 120/Fat:8 g/Protein:12 g/Carbs: 1 g

Easy Zucchini Beef Lasagna

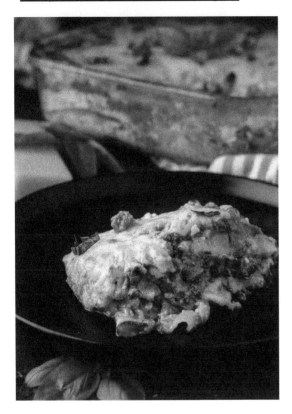

Prep time: 20 min

Cook time: 1 hour

Servings: 4

Ingredients 1 lb ground beef 2 large zucchinis, sliced lengthwise 3 cloves garlic 1 medium white onion, chopped 3 tomatoes, chopped Salt and black pepper to taste 2 tsp sweet paprika 1 tsp dried thyme 1 tsp dried basil 1 cup mozzarella cheese, shredded 1 tbsp olive oil Preheat the oven to 370°F.

Method: Heat the vegetable oil in an exceedingly frypan over medium heat. Cook the beef for 4 minutes while breaking any lumps as you stir. Top with onion, garlic, tomatoes, salt, paprika, and pepper. Stir and continue cooking for 5 minutes. Lay ⅓ of the zucchini slices in the baking dish. Top with ⅓ of the beef mixture and repeat the layering process two more times with the same quantities. Season with basil and thyme. Sprinkle the mozzarella cheese on top and tuck the baking dish in the oven. Bake for 35 minutes. Remove the lasagna and let it rest for 10 minutes before serving.

Nutritional info per serve:: Kcal 344, Fat 17.8g, Net Carbs 2.9g, Protein 40.4g

Broccoli and Bacon Bowls

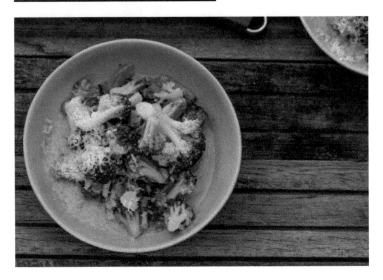

Prep time: 15 minutes

Cook time: 7 minutes

Servings: 4

Ingredients: 1 cup broccoli florets, 1 spring onion, sliced 5 oz bacon, fried chopped, 5 oz Monterey Jack cheese, grated 1 tablespoon ricotta cheese 1 tablespoon fresh parsley, chopped ½ teaspoon chili powder 1 cup water, for cooking

Method: Pour water in the pan and bring it to boil. Add broccoli florets and boil them for 7 minutes. After this, remove broccoli from the water and transfer it in the big bowl. In the separated bowl, mix fresh parsley, chili powder, and ricotta cheese. Melt the mixture and add in the broccoli. Then add Monterey Jack cheese, spring onion, and bacon. Shake the meal well and transfer in the serving bowls.

Nutritional info per serve: Calories 344, Fat 26, Fiber 1, Carbs 4, Protein 23.1

Beef Meatballs with Onion Sauce

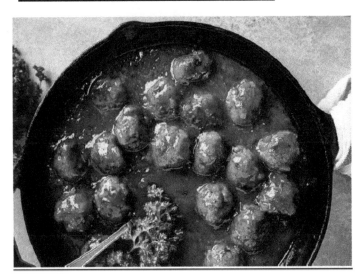

Prep time: 7 minutes

Cook time 32 minutes

Servings: 4

Ingredients: 1 lb ground beef Salt and black pepper to taste ½ tsp garlic powder 1 ¼ tbsp coconut aminos 1 cup beef stock ¾ cup almond flour 1 tbsp fresh parsley, chopped 1 tbsp dried onion flakes 1 onion, sliced 2 tbsp butter ¼ cup sour cream

Methods: In a bowl, mix the beef, salt, garlic powder, almond flour, onion flakes, parsley, 1 tbsp coconut aminos, and pepper. Form balls. Place them on a greased baking sheet. Bake in the oven for 20 minutes at 370°F. Heat the butter in an exceedingly pan over medium heat. Stir within the onion and cook for three minutes. Pour in the beef stock, sour cream, and remaining coconut aminos and bring to a simmer. Season with salt and pepper and cook for 3-4 minutes until the sauce thickens. Put the sauce over the meatballs and serve.

Nutritional info per serve: Kcal 435, Fat 23g, Net Carbs 6g, Protein 32g

Smoked Whitefish Salad

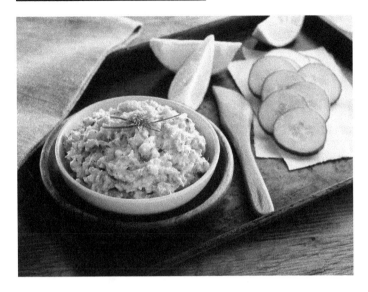

Prep time: 25 minutes

Cook time: 3 hours

Servings: 3

Ingredients: 1 Ib. smoked whitefish, chunked, ½ cup celery, diced ½ cup red onion, diced ½ cup crème, fraise, ½ cup cream cheese 1 tablespoon fresh chives, 1 tablespoon dill, 2 teaspoons lemon juice

Methods: Place the whitefish in a bowl with celery and red onion Toss to combine. If you'd sort of a less chunky dish, you'll place the ingredients in an exceedingly kitchen appliance and pulse till lessened into smaller items. In another bowl, mix the crème fraise, cheese, chives, dill, and lemon juice; add Salt and pepper to style if desired. mix till

creamy. Add the cream mixture to the whitefish and blend till emulsified. cowl and refrigerate for 2 hours before serving.

Nutritional info per serve: Kcal 386.7/ Fat: 12.2 g/Protein: 31 g/ Carbs: 4.2

Stuffed Peppers with Ground Beef and Cheese

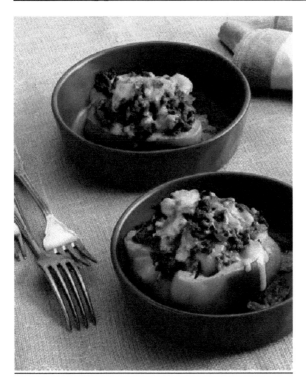

Prep time: 5 minutes

Cook Time: 30 min

Servings: 6

Ingredients: 1 oz. butter, for greasing 4 green bell peppers, cut lengthwise and discard the seeds. 4 tbsp extra-virgin olive oil, divided 1 yellow onion, chopped 2 garlic cloves, chopped oz. boeuf two tsp flavouring two tsp ground cumin seven oz. tomatoes salt and pepper 8 oz. shredded cheddar cheese, divided 8 oz. sour cream 4 oz. spinach

Methods: Preheat the oven to 400°F. Grease a baking dish with butter. Place the peppers in the baking dish. Drizzle 2 tbsp. of the olive oil. Heat the remaining of the olive oil in a frying pan, over medium heat. Add the onions and garlic and cook for about 40 seconds or until tender. Add the bottom beef and cook till soft-bo through. Add the chili, cumin, and tomatoes. Simmer for about 10 minutes. Add salt and pepper to taste. Remove from heat. Add the chess and stir to combine. Stuff the peppers with ground-beef mixture add the cheese on top. Bake for concerning twenty minutes or till the cheese has thawed.

Nutritional info per serve: Kcal 574 / Fat 40 g. / Carbs 3 g. / Protein 26 g.

Shrimp and Avocado Salad

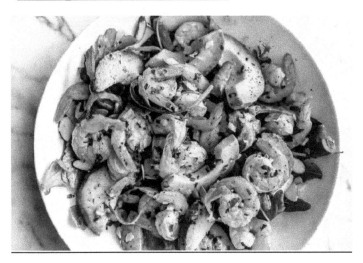

Prep time: 12 minutes

Cook time: 8 minutes

Servings: 4

Ingredients: 1-pound shrimps, peeled 1 avocado, chopped 1 tablespoon sesame oil, 1 teaspoon sesame seeds ½ teaspoon chili powder ½ cup fresh spinach ½ teaspoon coconut oil

Methods: Melt the coconut oil in the skillet and add shrimps. Sprinkle them with chili powder and roast for 2 minutes per side. Then transfer the shrimps in the salad bowl and add all remaining ingredients. Shake the salad well.

Nutritional info per serve: Kcal 278/ Fat 16.1/ Fiber 3.7,/Carbs 6.5/ Protein 27.1

Ribeye Steak with Shitake Mushrooms

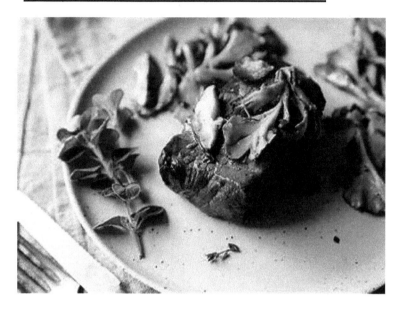

Prep time: 5 minutes

Cook time: 20 minutes

Servings: 4

Ingredients: 1 lb ribeye steaks, 1 tbsp butter, 2 tbsp olive oil, 1 cup shitake mushrooms, sliced Salt and black pepper to taste, 2 tbsp fresh parsley, chopped

Methods: Heat the olive oil in a pan over medium heat. Rub the steaks with salt and black pepper and cook about 4 minutes per side; reserve. Melt the butter in the pan and cook the shitakes for 4 minutes. Scatter the parsley over and pour the mixture over the steaks to serve.

Nutritional info per serve:: Kcal 478/Fat: 31g/Carbs: 3g/Protein: 33g

Mexican Beef Chili

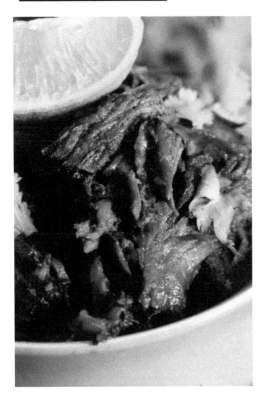

Prep time: 10 minutes

Cook time: 30 minutes

Servings: 4

Ingredients: 15 oz canned tomatoes with green chilies, chopped 1 onion, chopped 2 tbsp olive oil 1 ½ lb ground beef 1 cup beef broth 1 tbsp tomato paste ½ cup pickled jalapeños, chopped 1 tsp chipotle chili paste 2 garlic cloves, minced 3 celery stalks, chopped 2 tbsp coconut aminos Salt and black pepper to taste ½ tsp cayenne pepper 1 tsp cumin 1 bay leaf 1 tbsp fresh cilantro, chopped

Methods: Heat the olive oil in a pan over medium heat. Add in the onion, celery, garlic, ground beef, black pepper, and salt and cook until the meat browns, about 6-8 minutes. Stir in jalapeños, tomato paste, canned tomatoes with green chilies, salt, bay leaf, cayenne pepper, coconut aminos, chipotle chili paste, beef broth, and cumin. Cook for 30 minutes. Remove and discard the bay leaf. Serve sprinkled with cilantro.

Nutritional info per serve:: Kcal 437/ Fat 26g/Carbs 5g/Protein 17g

Roasted Pork with Lemon & Rosemary

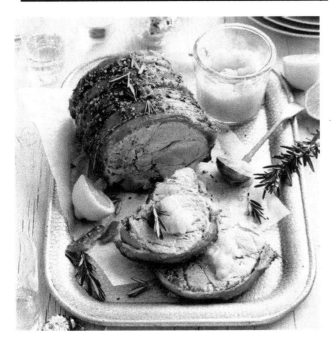

Prep time: 10 minutes

CookTime: 45 minutes

Servings: 4

Ingredients 24 oz. pork tenderloin 1 tbsp garlic, minced 1 tsp coriander, crushed 3 tbsp extra-virgin olive oil 1/2 tbsp lemon juice 1/2 tsp grated lemon zest 2 tbsp fresh thyme 1 1/2 tsps dried rosemary 1 1/2 tsps dried ground sage 3 tsps salt 1/2 tsps ground black pepper

Methods: Preheat the oven to 425°F. Line the baking sheet with associate tin foil. Mix the garlic, coriander, olive oil, lemon juice, lemon zest, thyme, rosemary, sage, salt, and pepper in a small bowl and mix well. Pour the sauce mixture over the pork and rub in. Place the pork on a baking sheet. Bake for about 40 minutes or until cooked through and browned. Let cool before slicing. Remove from the oven. Add the sauce on the pork and serve.

Nutritional info per serve: Kcal 321 / Fat 20 g/Carbs 0 g./Pro 28 g.

Beef Taco Salad

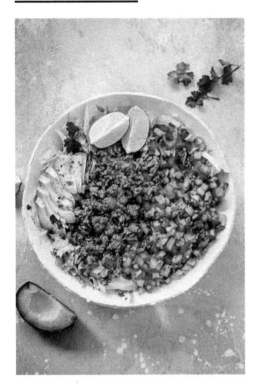

Prep time: 5 min

Cook Time: 25 min

Servings: 2

Ingredients: 2 romaine lettuce, chopped 9 oz. ground beef 1 ripe avocado 4 oz. salsa 4 oz. shredded mexican cheese 2 tbsp sour cream Seasonings 1 tbsp paprika 1 tsp garlic powder 1 tsp onion powder 1/2 tsp cayenne powder

Method: Start heating the pan on medium heat and then add coconut oil in it. Add the ground beef and cook until cooked through add in the seasoning and mix well. Placing the lettuce in a bowl and followed by the beef, avocado, salsa, sour cream and the cheese.

Nutritional info per serve: Kcal 585/Fat 53 g. / Carbs 8 g. /Pro 19 gr.

Delicious Lunch Pizza

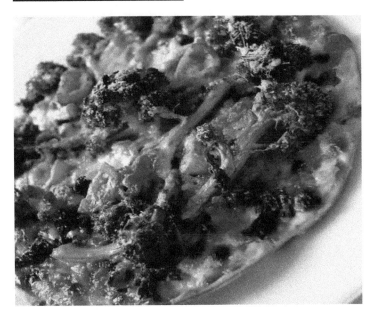

Prep time: 20 minutes

Cook time: 30 minutes

Servings: 4

Ingredients: 1 ¼ cup pizza cheese mix, shredded, , 1 tablespoon olive oil, 1 tablespoons ghee, 1 cup mozzarella cheese, shredded ¼ cup mascarpone cheese, 1 tablespoon heavy cream, 1 teaspoon garlic, minced Salt and black pepper to the taste, A pinch of lemon pepper, 1/3 cup broccoli florets, steamed, Some asiago cheese, shaved for serving **Methods:** Heat a pan with the oil over medium heat, add pizza pie cheese combine, and unfold into a circle.. Add mozzarella cheese and also spread it into a circle. Cook everything for 7 minutes and transfer to a plate. Heat the pan with the ghee over medium heat, add mascarpone cheese, cream, salt, pepper, lemon pepper, and garlic, stir and cook for 5 minutes. Drizzle half this combine over cheese crust. Add broccoli florets to the pan with the remainder of the cream cheese mix; stir and cook for one minute. Add this to the pizza, sprinkle asiago cheese at the end, and serve. Enjoy!

Nutritional info per serve: Kcal 270/Fat: 8 g/Pro:15g/Carbs: 2.5 gr

Special Fish Pie

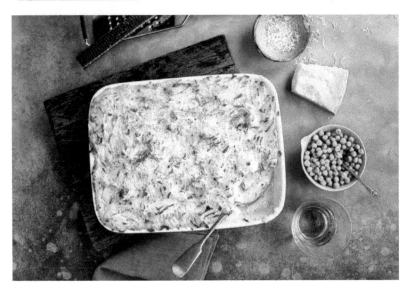

Prep time: 15 minutes

Cook time: 1 hour 20 minutes

Servings: 6

Ingredients: one purple onion, chopped , a pair of salmon fillets, skinless and take medium items , a pair of mackerel fillets, skinless and take medium items , three haddock fillets and take medium items, 2 bay leaves ¼ cup ghee , 1 cauliflower head, florets separated , 4 eggs , 4 cloves 1 cup whipping cream , ½ cup water, A pinch of nutmeg, ground , 1 teaspoon Dijon mustard, 1 cup cheddar cheese, shredded+ ½ cup cheddar cheese, shredded,   Some chopped parsley, Salt , Black pepper 4 tablespoons chives, chopped

Method: Put some water in a pan, add some salt, bring to a boil over medium heat, add eggs, cook them for 10 minutes, take off heat, drain, leave them to cool down down, peel, and cut them into quarters. Put water in another pot, bring to a boil, add cauliflower florets, cook for 10 minutes, drain them, transfer to your blender, add ¼ cup ghee, pulse well and transfer to a bowl. Put the cream and ½ cup water in a pan, add fish, toss to coat, and heat up over medium heat. Add onion, cloves, and bay leaves, bring to a boil, reduce heat and simmer for 10 minutes. Take off heat, transfer fish to a baking dish and leave aside. Return pan with fish sauce to heat, add nutmeg, stir and cook for 5 minutes. Take off heat, discard cloves and bay leaves, add one cup cheddar cheese and two tablespoons ghee and stir well. Place egg quarters on top of the fish in the baking dish. Add cream and cheese sauce over them, top with cauliflower mash, sprinkle the rest of the cheddar cheese, chives and parsley, introduce in the oven at 400 degrees F for 30 minutes. Leave the pie to cool down a bit before slicing and serving. Enjoy your meal.
Nutritional info per serve:: 370/ Fat: 38 g/ Pro: 32 g Carbs: 4.5 gr

Pancetta & Kale Pork Sausages

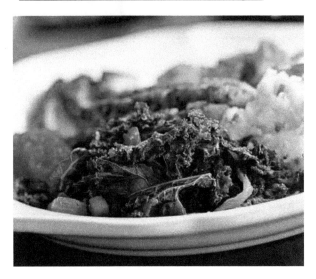

Prep time: 30 minutes

Servings: 4

Ingredients 2 cups kale 4 cups chicken broth 2 tbsp olive oil 1 cup heavy cream 3 pancetta slices, chopped ½ lb radishes, chopped 2 garlic cloves, minced Salt and black pepper to taste ½ tsp red pepper flakes 1 onion, chopped 1 ½ lb hot pork sausage, chopped

Method: heat the vegetable oil during a pot over medium heat. Stir in garlic, onion, pancetta, and sausage and cook for 5 minutes. Pour in the broth, radishes, and kale and simmer for 10 minutes. Add salt, red pepper, and black pepper. Add in the heavy cream, stir, and cook for about 5 minutes. Serve.

Nutritional info per serve: Kcal 386, Fat 29g, Net Carbs 5.4g, Pro 21g

Ketogenic Dessert Recipes

<u>Butter Truffles</u>

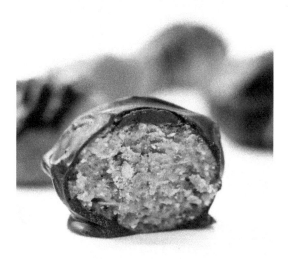

Prep time: 10 minutes

Cook time: 5 minutes

Servings: 10

Ingredients: 3 oz dark chocolate, chopped 2 tablespoons butter ⅔ cup coconut cream 2 tablespoons Erythritol ¼ teaspoon vanilla extract 1 teaspoon of cocoa powder

Methods: Melt the chocolate and mix it with butter. Add coconut cream, Erythritol, and vanilla extract. Then make the small balls (truffles) and coat them in the cocoa powder. Refrigerate the dessert for 10-15 minutes before serving.

Nutritional info per serve: Kcal 103/Fat 8.7/Fiber 0.7/ Carbs 6.1/Protein 1.1

Easy Coconut Mousse

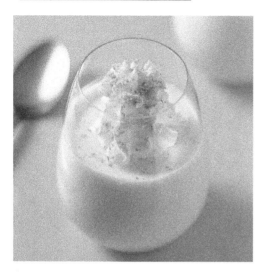

Prep time: 7 minutes

Cook time : 12 minutes

Servings: 6

Ingredients: 1/2 cup coconut milk A pinch of grated nutmeg 1 cup double cream 1/2 cup panela cheese 2 tablespoons powdered Erythritol 1/2 cup coconut creamer 1 ½ cups avocado, pitted, peeled and mashed

Methods: Warm the coconut milk and creamer over low heat. Remove from the heat. Stir in the avocado and nutmeg; continue to stir until everything is well incorporated. Add in the remaining ingredients. Beat using an electric mixer on medium-high speed. Place in your refrigerator until firm.Enjoy!

Nutritional info per serve 303 Calories; 30g Fat; 3.1g Carbs; 3.5g Protein; 2.7g Fiber

Vanilla Coconut Waffles

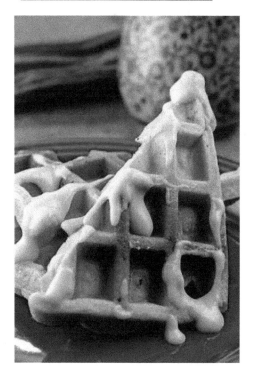

Prep time: 5 minutes

Cook Time: 15 min

Servings: 2

Ingredients: 1 tbsp coconut oil 1 egg, separated white and yolk 4 oz. almond flour 2 tbsp stevia 1/2 tsp baking powder 1/4 tsp Sea salt 2 tbsp peanut butter 2 tbsp coconut oil 2 oz. unsweetened coconut milk 1/2 tbsp grated coconut 1/2 tsp Vanilla extract

Methods: Preheat the waffle iron to high heat. Grease lightly with coconut oil. Add the egg white in a bowl and whisk to combine. Set aside. Add almond flour, stevia, baking powder, and salt in a bowl and combine well. Set aside. Add melted butter and peanut butter together and whisk together. Add the mixture to the dry flour bowl. Add the yolk, coconut milk, grated coconut and vanilla to the batter. Stir until smooth. Fold the egg whites into the batter and mix well until the batter is fluffy. Transfer half the batter into the greased waffle iron. Cook for about 5 minutes. Repeat with the remaining batter. Transfer to a plate and serve.

Nutritional info per serve: Kcal 384/ Fat 35 g. / Carbs 4 g. / Pro 10 g.

Basic Orange Cheesecake

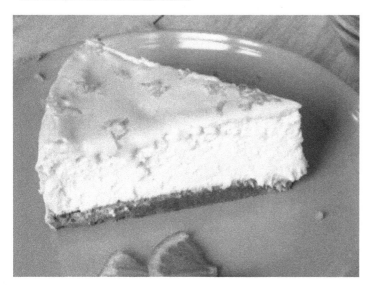

Prep time: quarter-hour

Cook time: ten minutes

Servings: twelve

Ingredients: Crust: one tablespoon Swerve, one cup almond flour, one stick butter, temperature, 1/2 cup sugarless coconut, sliced Filling: one teaspoon pulverized gelati n, a pair of tablespoons Swerve seventeen ounces cream cheese cream, a pair of tablespoons fruit crush

Methods: completely mix all the ingredients for the crust. Press the crust mixture into a gently lubricated baking dish. Let it fill in your icebox. Then, combine one cup of boiling water and gelatin till all are dissolved. Pour in one cup of cold water. Add Swerve, cream cheese cheese, and orange juice; mix till sleek and uniform. Pour the filling onto the ready crust. Serve and revel in your meal.

Nutritional information per serve: Kcals 150/Fat: thirteen g/Pro a pair of g /Carbs five gr

Pecan Brownies

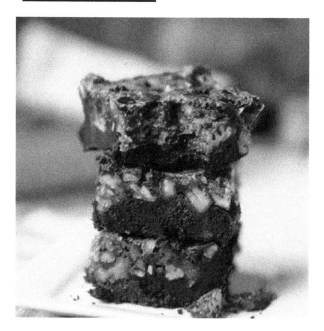

Prep time: 20 minutes

Cook time: 30 minutes

Servings:4

Ingredients: 3 eggs, beaten 2 tablespoons cocoa powder 2 teaspoons Erythritol ½ cup coconut flour 2 pecans, chopped ½ cup of coconut milk

Method: In the mixing bowl, mix eggs with cocoa powder, Erythritol, coconut flour, pecans, and coconut milk. Stir the mixture until smooth and pour it into the brownie mold. Flatten the surface of the brownie batter if needed. Bake it at 360F for 25 minutes. When the brownie is cooked, cut it into bars.

Nutritional info per serving: Kcal 178/Fat 16/Carbs 5.4/Pro 6.3

Chocolate Chip Cookies

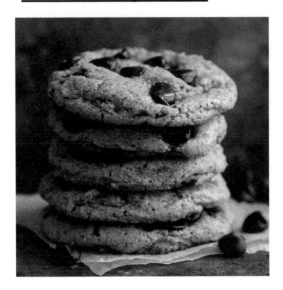

Prep time: 5 minutes

Cook Time: 15 minutes

Servings: 4

Ingredients:1 cup butter, softened 2 cups swerve brown sugar 3 eggs 2 cups almond flour 2 cups unsweetened chocolate chips Preheat oven to 350°F.

Method: Line a baking sheet with parchment paper. Whisk the butter and sugar with a hand mixer for 3 minutes or until light and fluffy. Add the eggs one at a time, and scrape the sides as you whisk. Mix in almond flour at low speed until well combined. Fold in the chocolate chips. Scoop 3 tablespoons each on the baking sheet, creating spaces between each mound, and bake for 15 minutes to swell and harden. Remove, cool, and serve.

Nutritional info per serve: Kcal 317,/Fat 27g/ Carbs 8.9g/Pro 6.3g

Chocolate Avocado Mousse

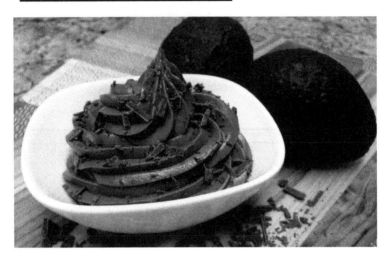

Prep time: 5 minutes

Cook Time: 16 min

Servings: 4

Ingredients: 4 ripe avocados 4 oz. unsweetened cocoa powder 4 oz. chocolate chips melted 8 tbsp coconut milk 1 tsp vanilla extract 1 tsp salt stevia

Method: Add all the ingredients to a food blender and blend until smooth. Transfer to cups and serve.

Nutritional info per serve: Kcal 395/Fat 40 g./Carbs 10 g./ Pro 9 g.

Strawberry Pie

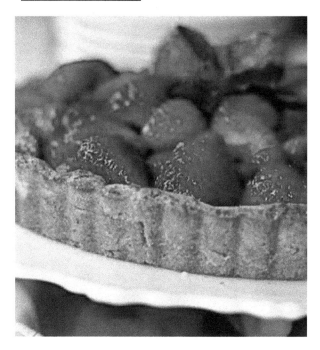

Prep time: a pair of hours

Cook time: twenty minutes

Servings: ten

Ingredients: For the crust: one cup coconut, chopped one cup helianthus seeds ¼ cup butter A pinch of salt For the filling: one teaspoon gelatin eight ounces cheese four ounces strawberries a pair of tablespoons water ½ tablespoon juice ¼ teaspoon stevia ½ cup cream eight ounces strawberries, cut for serving sixteen ounces cream for serving

Method: In your kitchen appliance, combine helianthus seeds with coconut, a pinch of salt, and butter and stir well. place this into a lubricated springform pan and press well on an all-time low. Heat a pan with the water over medium heat, add gelatin, stir till it dissolves, and begin the warmth and leave aside to cool down. Add this to your kitchen appliance, combine with four ounces strawberries, cheese, juice, stevia, and mix well. Add ½ cup cream, stir well, and unfold this over crust. prime with eight ounces strawberries and sixteen ounces cream and confine the icebox for two hours before slicing and serving. Serve and revel in your meal.

Nutritional data per serve: Kcal 235/Fat: eighteen g/Pro: forty two g Carbs: half-dozen gr

Chocolate Bark with Almonds

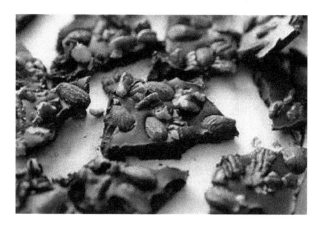

Prep time: 5 minutes

Cook time: cooling time

Servings: 12

Ingredients: ½ cup toasted almonds, chopped ½ cup butter 10 drops stevia ¼ tsp salt ½ cup unsweetened coconut flakes 4 oz dark chocolate **Method:** Melt together the butter and chocolate, in the microwave, for 90 seconds. Remove and stir in stevia. Line a cookie sheet with waxed paper and spread the chocolate evenly. Scatter the almonds on high, coconut flakes, and sprinkle with salt. Refrigerate for one hour.

Nutritional info per serve: Kcal 161/Fat: 15.3g/Carbs: 1.9g/Pro: 1.9g

Breakfast Yogurt Parfait

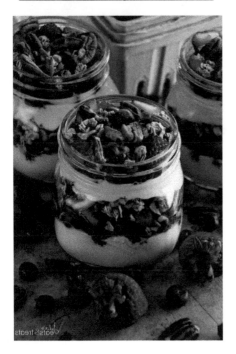

Prep time: 1 min

Cook Time: 5 min

Servings: 1

Ingredients: 2 tbsp pecan, chopped 2 oz. blueberries 8 oz. yogurt strawberry

Method: Layer pecan, blueberries and yogurt in a glass cup And serve.

Nutritional info per serve Kcal 185 / Fat 17 g. / Carbs 5 g. / Pro 14 g.

Coconut Pancakes

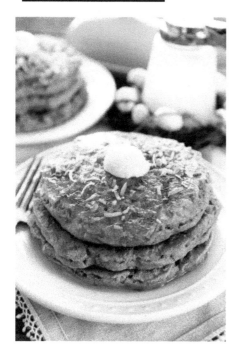

Prep time: 10 minutes

Cook time: 15 minutes

Servings: 4

Ingredients: ½ cup almond flour , ½ cup coconut flour , 1 tablespoon coconut shred, 1 tablespoon Erythritol, 1 teaspoon baking powder • ½ teaspoon vanilla extract, 1 tablespoon avocado oil, ½ cup heavy cream

Method: Heat the skillet and pour avocado oil inside. Then mix all remaining ingredients in the bowl, stir it until you get a smooth batter. Pour the small amount of batter in the hot skillet and flatten it in the shape of a pancake. Roast the pancake on medium heat for 1 minute per side. Repeat the same steps with all remaining batter.

Nutritional info per serve: Calories 216, Fat 15.4, Fiber 7.9, Carbs 18.5, Protein 5.4

Sesame Lemon Mug Cake

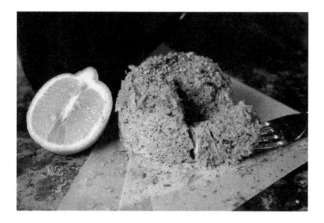

Prep time: 2 min

Cook Time: 10 min

Servings: 1

Ingredients: 1 egg 2 tbsp butter 2 tbsp almond flour 1/2 tsp baking powder 1 tbsp sesame seed 1 tsp lemon juice 1/4 tsp pepper salt

Method: Mix all ingredients together. Add in the microwave and cook for about 75 seconds over high heat. Take the mug cake out. Add sesame seeds and serve.

Nutritional info per serve:Kcal 393 /Fat 32 g. /Carbs 4 g. / Pro 10 g.

Keto Snacks and appetizers

Chili Biscuits

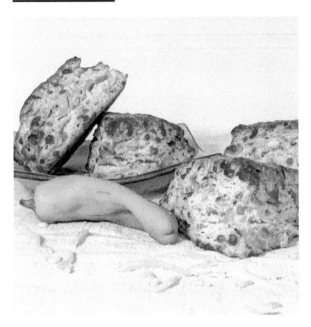

Prep time: 20 minutes

Cook time: 20 minutes

Servings: 8

Ingredients: 1 cup almond flour 1 teaspoon chili powder 1 teaspoon smoked paprika 3 teaspoons coconut oil 1 tablespoon sesame oil

Method: Brush the baking pan with sesame oil. Then mix all remaining ingredients in the mixing bowl and knead the dough. Make the small biscuits and put them in the baking pan. Bake the meal ta 360F for 15 minutes.

Nutritional info per serve: Kcal 51, Fat 5.2, Fiber 0.6, Carbs 1.1, Protein 0.8

Italian Cheese Crisps

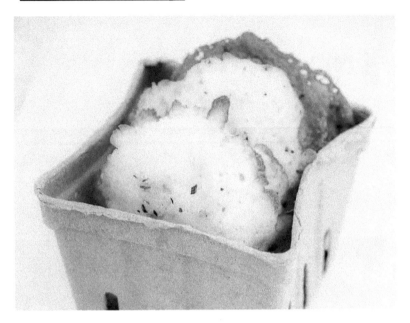

Prep time: twelve minutes

Cook time: zero minutes

Servings: three

Ingredients: one cup sharp cheddar, grated 1/4 teaspoon ground black pepper, 1/2teaspoon cayenne pepper, one teaspoon Italian seasoning

Method: begin by preheating associate degree kitchen appliance to four hundred degrees F. Line a baking sheet with parchment paper. combine all of them on top of ingredients till well combined. Then, place tablespoon-sized loads of the mixture onto the ready baking sheet. Bake at the preheated kitchen appliance for eight minutes till the edges begin to brown. enable the cheese crisps to chill slightly. Then, place them on paper towels to empty the surplus fat. Finally, Enjoy!

Nutritional information per serve: Kcal one30/Fat8 g/ Pro12 g/Carbs: 1.5 gr

Seed Crackers & Guacamole

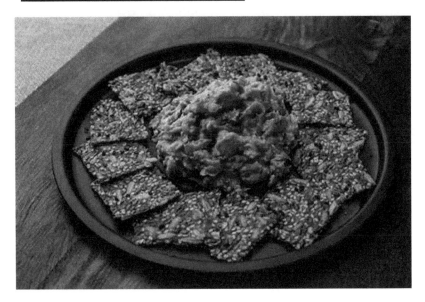

Prep time: twenty minutes

Cook Time: fifty min

Servings: four

Ingredients: two oz. Chia seeds two oz. benne seeds two oz. Helianthus seeds 1/2 tbsp herb combine seasoning 1/2 tsp salt eight oz. water dip 1/2 mashed avocado Juice of [*fr1] a lime Pinch of ocean salt

Method: heat the kitchen appliance to 175°C. cowl a baking sheet with parchment paper Add all the seeds with water and seasonings. Let the mixture sit for five minutes. unfold the seed mixture equally till flat. Bake for half-hour and take away from the kitchen appliance, take away squares. Flip and bake for an additional quarter-hour. Add all the dip ingredients in an exceedingly bowl to mix and mash till swish.

Nutritional data per serve: Kcal fifteen4 / Fat 15 g. / Carbs four g. / Pro 2g.

Rich Keto Grits with Hemp

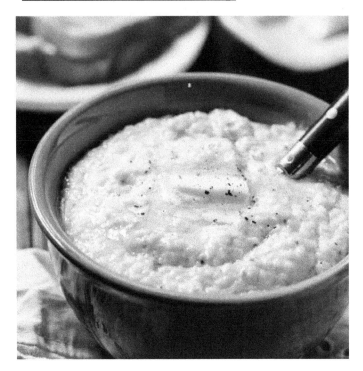

Prep time: five minutes

Cook time: twenty minutes

Servings: four

Ingredients: 1/4 cup hemp hearts two tablespoons butter, softened one teaspoon coconut extract 1/4 teaspoon coarse salt eight walnuts, shredded four eggs, gently whisked 1/4 cup flax seed, freshly ground two teaspoons liquid Monk fruit 1/4 teaspoon pinch fleawort husk powder

Method: Mel the butter in an exceedingly sauté pan over medium-low heat. Add within the remaining ingredients and still cook till the mixture starts

to boil. take away from heat and stir within the shredded walnuts; stir to mix.

Nutritional data per   serve: 405   Calories;   37g   Fat; vi.6g Carbs; fourteen.8g Protein; two.3g Fiber

Tortilla Chips

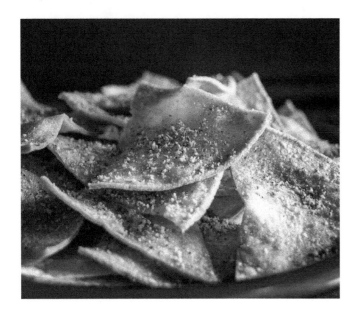

Prep time: quarter-hour

Cook time: eighteen minutes

Servings: half-dozen

Ingredients: For the tortillas: a pair of teaspoons oil one cup flax seed meal a pair of tablespoons Spanish psyllium husk powder ¼ teaspoon xanthan gum one cup water ½ teaspoon flavourer three teaspoons coconut flour For the chips: half-dozen linseed tortillas Salt Black pepper three tablespoons edible fat recent condiment for serving cream for serving

Method: during a bowl, combine linseed meal with Spanish psyllium powder, olive oil, xanthan gum, water, and flavourer and blend till you get an elastic dough. unfold coconut flour on an operating surface. Divide dough into six items, place each bit on the operating surface, roll into a circle and cut every into six items. Heat a pan with the edible fat over medium-high heat, add flapjack chips, and cook for two minutes on both sides and transfer to paper towels. place flapjack chips during a bowl, season with salt and pepper, and serve with some recent condiment and cream on the aspect. Serve your dish.

Nutritional data per serve:

Kcal: thirty Fat: three g/Pro: seven g/Carbs: .5 g

Eggplant Parmesan

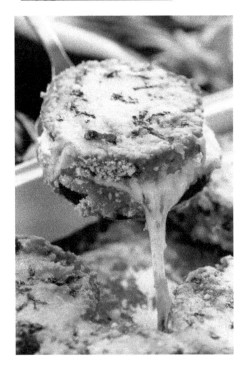

Prep time: 20 minutes

Cook Time: 1 hr

Servings: 5

Ingredients: 1 large eggplant ,sliced 16 oz. mozzarella cheese thinly slices 4 oz. shredded parmesan cheese 2 oz. butter 2 large cloves garlic, minced 28 oz. tomatoes crushed 1/4 tsp red pepper flakes, crushed 2 oz. basil, chopped 2 oz. coconut flour 2 eggs, beaten Salt 4 tbsp olive oil

Method: Preheat the oven at 350 °F (175°C). Add butter and the garlic in a skillet and place over medium heat until the garlic starts to brown, add the tomatoes, red pepper flakes, and a pinch of salt. Bring to a simmer and stir occasionally for about 6 minutes until the sauce thickens. Remove from heat and add the basil and stir to combine. Heat a sheet pan in the oven for about 10 minutes. Sprinkle each side of the eggplant slices with salt. Dredge an eggplant slice in the coconut flour and dip in the egg. Repeat with the remaining eggplant. Remove the heated sheet pan from the oven and brush it with butter. Place the eggplant on the sheet pan. Bake for regarding ten minutes or till crisp and suntanned. . Flip the slices and continue baking for about 10 minutes more or until golden. Drizzle with the baked eggplant with tomato sauce, olive oil, mozzarella, and Parmesan. Bake for 20 minutes or until the cheese melts and browns. Top with basil before serving.

Nutritional info per serve: Kcal 429 / Fat 34 g. / Carbs 9 g. / Protein 16 g.

Cheese Roll Up

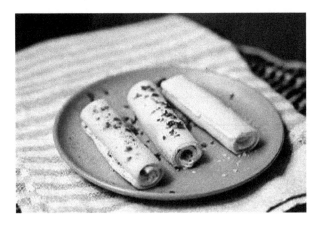

Prep time: 7 minutes

Cook Time: 7 minutes

Servings: 4

Ingredients 9 oz. shredded cheddar cheese 4 oz. butter 2 tsp parsley, chopped

Method: Place the cheese slices on a large cutting board. Slice butter with a cheese slicer Cover every cheese slice with butter. Roll up the cheese. Sprinkle chopped parsley on rolled up cheese and serve. **Nutritional info per serve:** Kcal 329 / Fat 46 g. / Carbs 3 g. / Pro 9gr

Fried Queso Snack

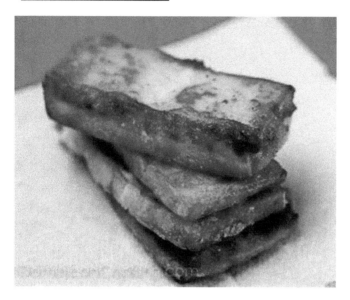

Prep time: 10 minutes

Cook time: 20 minutes

Servings: 6

Ingredients: 2 ounces olives, pitted and chopped, 5 ounces queso Blanco cubed and freeze for a couple of minutes A pinch of red pepper flakes 1 and ½ tablespoons olive oil

Method: Heat a pan with the oil over medium-high heat, add queso cubes and cook until the bottom melts a bit. Flip cubes with a spatula and sprinkle black olives on top. Leave cubes to cook a bit more, flip and sprinkle red pepper flakes and cook until they are crispy. Flip, cook on the other side until it's crispy as well, transfer to a cutting board, cut into small blocks and then serve as a snack.

Nutritional info per serve: Kcal: 530/Fat: 38 g/Pro 52 g/Carbs: 3.5 gr

Spinach Dip

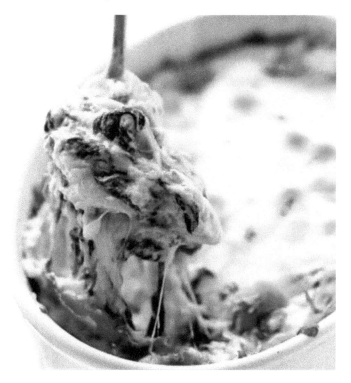

Prep time: 5 minutes

Cook time: 10 minutes

Servings: 6

Ingredients: 1 ½ cup spinach, chopped, 2 tablespoons cream cheese, 1 tablespoon coconut oil, ¼ cup Cheddar cheese, grated, ¼ cup heavy cream, ½ teaspoon chili powder

Method: Put all ingredients in the saucepan and carefully mix. Then cook the mixture on low heat for 10 minutes or until it starts to boil.

Blend the mixture with the help of the immersion blender and simmer for 2-3 minutes more.

Nutritional info per serve: KCal 70, Fat 6.9, Fiber 0.3, Carbs 0.7, Protein 1.8

Chicken Nuggets

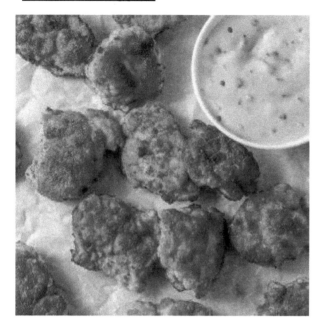

Prep time: ten minutes

Cook time: sixteen minutes

Servings: two

Ingredients: ½ cup coconut flour 1 egg 2 tablespoons garlic powder 2 chicken breasts, cubed Salt and black pepper to the taste ½ cup ghee

Method: In a bowl, mix garlic powder with coconut flour, salt, pepper, and stir. In another bowl, whisk the egg well. Dip chicken breast cubes in egg mix, then in the flour mix Heat a pan with the clarified butter over medium heat, drop chicken nuggets and cook them for five minutes on both sides. Transfer to paper towels, drain grease, and then serve them with some tasty ketchup on the side. Enjoy your meal.

Nutritional info per serve: Kcal: 7O/Fat: 3 g /Pro: 5 g/ Carbs 2 gr.

Pumpkin Muffins

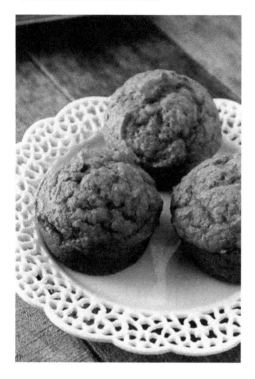

Prep time: quarter-hour

Cook time: twenty minutes

Servings: sixteen

Ingredients: ¼ cup edible seed butter ¾ cup pumpkin puree, two tablespoons oilseed meal, ¼ cup coconut flour½ cup erythritol, ½ teaspoon nutmeg, ground, one teaspoon cinnamon, ground, ½ teaspoon hydrogen carbonate, one egg ½ teaspoon leavening A pinch of salt

Method: during a bowl, combine butter with pumpkin puree and egg and mix well. Add oilseed meal, coconut flour, erythritol, hydrogen carbonate, baking powder, nutmeg, cinnamon, and a pinch of salt and stir well. Spoon this into a lubricated gem pan, introduce within the kitchen appliance at 350 degrees F and bake for a quarter-hour. Leave muffins to chill down and serve them as a snack. Enjoy!

Nutritional information per serve: Kcal 70/ Fat: 4g/Pro: twelve g/ Carbs: three gr

Grilled Garlic Parmesan Zucchini

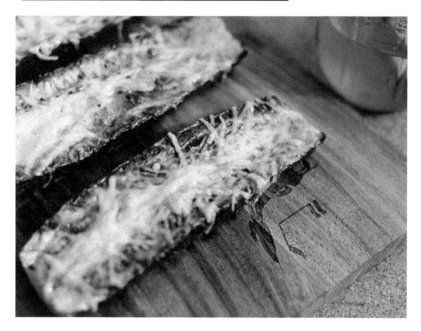

Prep time: 5 min

Cook Time: 35 min

Serving: 4

Ingredients: 3 zucchini 3 tbsp butter, melted salt, and pepper 2 cloves garlic, minced 1 tbsp fresh parsley, chopped 1 jalapeno sliced 4 oz. grated parmesan cheese

Method: Preheat the oven to 400°F. cowl a baking sheet with parchment paper. Cut the zucchini in half crosswise and slice each half into 3 slices lengthwise, making 6 slices per zucchini. Place the zucchini on a baking sheet. Brush the zucchini with butter. Season with salt and pepper. Sprinkle the garlic, parsley, jalapeno, and top with parmesan cheese. Bake for about 20 minutes or until the cheese has melted and the slices are cooked through. Serve warm.

Nutritional info per serve: Kcal 149 / Fat 12 g. / Carbs 4 g. / Pro 5gr

Conclusion

The main benefit of a ketogenic diet is its ability to lose weight quickly. Limiting enough carbohydrates to achieve ketosis also results in a significant reduction in body fat and an increase or maintenance of muscle mass. Studies show that long-term, low-carbohydrate diets can significantly reduce weight. Another primary reason people with diabetes eat a ketogenic diet is to lower and stabilize blood sugar. Carbohydrates are nutrients (macronutrients) that increase blood sugar the most. Since the ketogenic diet is deficient in carbohydrates, it reduces the high spikes in blood sugar. Several studies have shown that a ketogenic diet can lower blood pressure in overweight or type 2 diabetic people. In general, different ketogenic diets have various health benefits. We believe this book is a comprehensive collection of many keto recipes. It will show you everything you need to know about the ketogenic diet and get you started. In this book, you will know some of the best and most popular keto recipes in the world. I have accumulated these recipes for everyone! So, don't hesitate too much and start your new life as a follower of the Ketogenic diet! Get your hands on this special recipes collection and start cooking in this new, exciting and healthy way! Have a lot of fun and enjoy your Ketogenic diet!

CPSIA information can be obtained
at www.ICGtesting.com
Printed in the USA
BVHW051110260421
605873BV00019B/2384